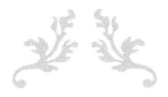

KETO DIET

FOR BEGINNERS

AFTER 50

Complete Guide For Senior Women To Ketogenic Diet And A Healthy Weight Loss | Including A 7 Tips For Succes For Beginners

CARLA RAMOS

TABLE OF CONTENTS

Introduction

Part of aging entails a deterioration in how we can function, but it doesn't have to collapse and separate. This is a tragic fact in our community for many seniors and elders above 50. The high-carb, processed diet that is often prescribed to this age group's people helps neither.

Keto foods have a high per caloric amount of protein. This is significant because the basal metabolic rate (the number of calories required daily for survival) is less for the elderly, but they require the same amount of nutrients as the younger ones.

A person 50+ would survive on fast foods much harder than a teen or 20-something whose body is resilient. That makes eating foods that are health-supporting and disease-fighting even more crucial for seniors. It can signify the difference between enjoying the golden years or spending them in pain and agony.

Much of the food preferred by older people (or delivered in a hospital or clinical setting) appears to be highly processed. It's very clear that the governments so commonly promoting high-carb diets isn't the best way to help our adult citizens and their long-term health. A diet low in carbohydrates and high in animal and plant fats are much healthier for improving insulin sensitivity, less cognitive losses, and better overall health.

Be patient and overcome those obstacles. At the end of the tunnel, the reward is too outstanding to give up on. Now about those hurdles ... you will run into them. And you will often entertain the thought of packing up and moving to some other program, perhaps you will go back to Weight Watchers or some other program that vents the freedom to eat "whatever you want" (as long as you control portions and count calories). But keep this in mind ... this goes against all the things we've just been thinking about. A fit and healthy person is not concerned about dieting, or about weight loss. But if you're always counting, tracking, or journalizing your calories and meals to weight loss, you will always be a struggling dietitian – one that's always afraid of relapse. You needn't be this person. Make that little sacrifice and get the reward that you've been looking for.

No matter your age, improving your chances of feeling and doing well for the rest of your life is never an awful idea. It's never too late to do better, even though our chances of preventing illness are higher the sooner we do. Ketosis for those over 50 can undo some damage, particularly for those who have spent several years not treating their bodies as well as they should have.

We're all growing older, and death is imminent. But the quality of life along the way is what we CAN manage to a degree. People are living longer now, but we get sicker also by following the majority's standard diet. This diet can help persons after 50 to boost their body's strength and endurance to survive in the later years of their lives, rather than being weak and lousy.

You'll also get more involved with health- and nutrition-related matters. It'll be only a matter of time before you feel amazing and full of energy. Slowly but gradually, you will turn yourself into the fit and the safe person I've been thinking about in mind and body. If you can stick with it for long enough (about 6-12 months), you can become this person altogether: safe, fit, and in total weight control. All come with time.

The basics of the keto diet

What Is A Keto Diet?

The keto diet is a very healthy and natural way to lose weight, but as with most new health regimens, there can be a rather lengthy period of change for some people–for some bodies, I should say. Truly, few will experience what we call the Keto-Flu during the beginning of the diet, and it typically lasts about a week, so don't be too concerned if you relate to these symptoms.

You all know that our body needs energy for its functioning and the energy sources come from carbohydrates, proteins, and fats. Owing to years of conditioning that a low-fat carbohydrate-rich diet is essential for good health, we have become used to depending on glucose (from carbohydrates) to get most of the energy that our body needs. Only when the amount of glucose available for energy generation decreases, does our body begin to break down fat for drawing energy to power our cells and organs. This is the express purpose of a ketogenic diet.

The primary aim of a ketogenic diet (called simply keto diet) is to convert your body into a fat-burning machine. Such a diet is loaded with benefits and is highly recommended by nutritional experts for the following end results:

- Natural appetite control
- Increased mental clarity

- Lowered levels of inflammation in the body system
- Improved stability in blood sugar levels
- Elimination or lower risk of heartburn
- Using natural stored body fat as the fuel source
- Weight loss

The effects listed are just some of the numerous effects that take place when a person embarks on a ketogenic diet and makes it a point to stick to it. A ketogenic diet consists of meals with low carbohydrates, moderate proteins, and high-fat content. The mechanism works like this: when we drastically reduce the intake of carbohydrates, our body is compelled to convert fat for releasing energy. This process of converting fats instead of carbohydrates to release energy is called ketosis.

How Does the Ketogenic Diet Work?

The time has come for you to get the answer to the question that has been lingering in your mind from the time you heard about the keto diet; 'how does a keto diet work?'

Here is how.

The power behind the Ketogenic diet's ability to help you lose weight and have better health comes from one simple action that the diet initiates in your body once you start following it. This simple action is how the keto diet changes your metabolism from burning carbohydrates for energy to burning fats for energy.

What does that have to do with weight loss and better health? Let me break it down for you.

- Burning carbohydrate for energy

Most of the food we eat follow the food pyramid recommended by the USDA some few decades ago. The pyramid puts carbohydrates at the bottom of the pyramid and fats at the top of the pyramid, which essentially means that carbohydrates form the bulk of the foods we eat, as shown below:

What many of us don't know is that when you consume a diet that is high in carbohydrates, two things normally happen.

- One, your body takes the just consumed carbohydrates and converts them into glucose which is the easiest molecule that your body can convert to use as energy (glucose is your body's primary source of energy, as it gets chosen over any other energy source in your body).

- Secondly, your body produces insulin for the sole purpose of it moving the glucose from your bloodstream into your cells where it can be used as energy.

There is more that goes unnoticed though:

Since your body gets its energy from glucose (which is mostly in huge amounts owing to the fact that we eat lots of high carbs food 3-6 times a day), it doesn't need any other source of energy. In fact, many are the times when glucose is in excess, something that prompts the body to convert dietary glucose into glycogen to be stored in the liver and muscle cells. What this simple explanation means is that with a high carb diet, your body is essentially in what we refer to as a fat-storing mode. It stores this excess fat so that it can use it when starved from its primary source of energy; glucose. Unfortunately, since we don't give ourselves enough breaks from food, we end up being in this constant fat-storing mode that ultimately causes weight gain.

• Burning fats for energy

As you now know, the Ketogenic diet is a low carb, high fat, and moderate protein diet. So, when you start following a Ketogenic diet, what typically happens is, your intake of carbohydrates is kept at a low. In other words, it inverts the USDA food pyramid I mentioned earlier, something that literally 'inverts/reverses' the effects of a high carb diet. How exactly does it do that?

Well, when you limit your carb intake greatly, you starve the body of its primary source of energy, something that initiates the process that the body has always been preparing for through its energy storage processes. More specifically, the body starts by metabolizing glycogen with the help of glucagon hormone (the process takes place in the liver). And with support from the human growth hormone, cortisol, and catecholamines (norepinephrine to be more specific), the body starts releasing fatty acids for use as energy in different body parts. But since fatty acids cannot be used by every cell in the body, the body is also forced to transport some of the fatty acids to the liver where they are broken down in a series of metabolic processes known as ketosis to produce three ketone bodies. Therefore, Ketosis is a natural process that your body activates when your energy intake is low for the purpose of helping you to survive. The three ketones that are formed when fatty acids are converted are:

- Acetone.
- Beta-hydroxybutyric acid (BHB)
- Acetoacetate (AcAc)

Many of your body cells (including the brain cells) can use BHB for energy, as it is water-soluble, something that makes it very much like glucose in that it can cross the blood-brain barrier. The more ketones the body cells use for energy, the more fat you are burning and ultimately, the more weight you stand to gain. Keep in mind that you are also taking lots of dietary fats. The reason for taking lots of dietary fats is to fill you up fast, make you stay full for longer and accustom the body cells to using fatty acids and ketones for energy so that when the deficit created by dietary fats kicks in (because you are unlikely to eat so many fats to the point of meeting your body's energy requirements- unless you are gluttonous), you begin burning stored body fat immediately, as opposed to starting with glycogen. Moderate intake of protein also helps you to get filled fast and to stay full for longer. Keeping your protein intake moderate is therefore vital, as any excess may end up causing you to get out of ketosis, as excess protein may be metabolized to glucose in a process known as gluconeogenesis. This essentially means a Ketogenic diet makes your body a fat-burning machine, as it relies primarily on fats (both dietary and stored body fat – though you want to get your body to burn as much of the stored boy fat as possible).

Ketosis helps you get rid of excessive fats in your body, which not only reduces your weight in an immense way but also betters your health by protecting you from various diseases as you will see.

To attain ketosis, you know that your intake of fats should be high, intake of carbs low and intake of proteins moderate. But what exactly does high, low and moderate translate to in calorie terms? In simpler terms, in what ratios should you take carbs, fats, and proteins? This gives rise to several types/approaches/schools of thought regarding the ratios:

Who invented this diet?

The ketogenic diet traces its roots to the treatment of epilepsy. Surprisingly this goes all the way back to 500 BC, when ancient Greeks observed that fasting or eating a ketogenic diet helped reduce epileptic seizures. In modern times, the ketogenic diet was reintroduced in the practice of medicine to treat children with epilepsy.

What is Ketosis?

Ketosis is a metabolic state where the body is efficiently using fat for energy. In a regular diet, carbohydrates produce glucose, which is used to provide energy. Glucose is stored in the body in fat cells that travel via the bloodstream. People gain weight when there is fatter stored than being used as energy.

Glucose is formed through the consumption of sugar and starch. Namely carbohydrates. The sugars may be in the form of natural sugars from fruit or milk, or they may be formed from processed sugar. Starches like pasta, rice or starchy vegetables like potatoes and corn, form glucose as well. The body breaks down the sugars from these foods into glucose. Glucose and insulin combined to help to carry glucose into the bloodstream so the body can use glucose as energy. The glucose that is not used is stored in the liver and muscles.

In order for the body to supply ketones for use as fuel, the body must use up all the reserves of glucose. In order to do this, there must be a condition of the body of low starvation carbohydrates, passing, or strenuous exercise. A very low carb diet, the production of ketones what her to feel the body and brain.

Ketones are produced from the liver when there is not enough glucose in the body to provide energy. When insulin levels are low, and there is not enough glucose or sugar in the bloodstream, fat is released from fat cells and travels in the blood to the liver. The liver processes the fat into ketones. Ketones are released into the bloodstream to provide fuel for the body and increase the body's metabolism. Ketones are formed under conditions of starvation, fasting, or a diet low in carbohydrates.

Benefits and side effects

Benefits Ketogenic diet

Reduction of risk of heart disease

Triglycerides, fat molecules in your body, have close links with heart disease. They are directly proportional as the more the number of triglycerides, the higher your chances of suffering from heart disease. You can reduce the number of free triglycerides in your body by reducing the number of carbohydrates, as is in the keto diets.

Reduces chances of having high blood pressure

Weight loss and blood pressure have a close connection; thus, since you are losing weight while on the keto diet, it will affect your blood pressure.

Fights type 2 diabetes

Type two diabetes develops as a result of insulin resistance. This is a result of having huge amounts of glucose in your system, with the keto diet this is not a possibility due to the low carbohydrate intake.

Increases the production of HDL

High-density lipoprotein is referred to as good cholesterol. It is responsible for caring calories to your liver, thus can be reused. High fat and low carbohydrate diets increase the production of HDL in your body, which also reduces your chances of getting heart disease. Low-density lipoprotein is referred to as bad cholesterol.

Suppresses your appetite

It is a strange but true effect of the keto diet. It was thought that this was a result of the production of ketones but this was proven wrong as a study taken between people on a regular balanced diet and some on the keto diet and their appetites were generally the same. It, however, helps to suppress appetite as it is it has a higher fat content than many other diets. Food stays in the stomach for longer as fat and is digested slowly, thus provides a sense of fullness. On top of that, proteins promote the secretion of cholecystokinin, which is a hormone that aids in regulating appetite. It is also believed that the ketogenic diet helps to suppress your appetite by continuous blunting of appetite. There is increased appetite in the initial stages of the diet, which decreases over time.

Changes in cholesterol levels

This is kind of on the fence between good and bad. This is because the ketogenic diet involves a high fat intake which makes people wonder about the effect on blood lipids and its potential to increase chances of heart disease and strokes, among others. Several major components play a lead role in determining this, which is: LDL, HDL, and blood triglyceride levels. Heart disease correlates with high levels of LDL and cholesterol. On the other hand, high levels of HDL are seen as protection from diseases caused by cholesterol levels. The impacts of the diet on cholesterol are not properly known. Some research has shown that there is no change in cholesterol levels while others have said that there is change. If you stay in deep ketosis for a very long period of time, your blood lipids will increase, but you will have to go through some negative effects of the ketogenic diet which will be corrected when the diet is over. If a person does not remain following the diet strictly for ten years, he/she will not experience any cholesterol problems. It is difficult to differentiate the difference between diet and weight loss in general. The effect of the ketogenic diet on cholesterol has been boiled down to if you lose fat on the ketogenic diet then your cholesterol levels will go down, and if you don't lose fat, then your cholesterol levels will go up. Strangely, women have a larger cholesterol level addition than men, while both are on a diet. As there is no absolute conclusion on the effect of the ketogenic diet on cholesterol, you are advised to have your blood lipid levels constantly checked for any bad effects. Blood lipid levels should be checked before starting the diet and about eight weeks after starting. If repeated results show a worsening of lipid levels, then you should abandon the diet or substitute saturated fats with unsaturated fats.

Risk of a ketogenic diet

Low energy levels

When available, the body prefers to use carbohydrates for fuel as they burn more effectively than fats. General drop-in energy level is a concern raised by many dieters due to the lack of carbohydrates. Studies have shown that it causes orthostatic hypotension which causes lightheadedness. It has come to be known that these effects can be avoided by providing enough supplemental nutrients like sodium. Many of the symptoms can be prevented by providing 5 grams of sodium per day. Most times, fatigue disappears after a few weeks or even days, if fatigue doesn't disappear, then you should add a small number of carbohydrates to the diet as long as ketosis is maintained. The diet is not recommended when carrying out high-intensity workouts, weight training, or high-intensity aerobic exercise as carbohydrates are an absolute requirement but are okay for low-intensity exercise.

Effects on the brain

It causes increased use of ketones by the brain. The increased use of ketones, among other reasons, result in the treating of childhood epilepsy. As a result of the changes that occur, the concern over the side effects, including permanent brain damage and short-term memory loss, has been raised. The origin of these concerns is difficult to understand. The brain is powered by ketones in the absence of glucose. Ketones are normal energy sources and not toxic as the brain creates enzymes, during fetal growth, that helps us use them. Epileptic children, though not the perfect examples, show some insight into the effects of the diet on the brain in the long term. There is no negative effect in terms of cognitive function. There is no assurance that the diet cannot have long term dietary effects, but no information proves that there are any negative effects. Some people feel they can concentrate more when on the ketogenic diet, while others feel nothing but fatigue. This is as a result of differences in individual physiology. There are very few studies that vaguely address the point on short term memory loss. This wore off with the continuation of the study.

Kidney stones and kidney damage

As a result of the increased workload from having to filter ketones, urea, and ammonia, as well as dehydration concerns of the potential for kidney damage or passing kidney stones have been raised. The high protein nature of the ketogenic diet raises the alarms of individuals who are concerned with potential kidney damage. There is very little information that points to any negative effects of the diet on kidney function or the development of kidney stones. There is a low incidence of small kidney stones in epileptic children; this may be as a result of the state of deliberate dehydration that the children are put at instead of the ketosis state itself. Some short term research shows no change in kidney function or increased incidents of kidney stones either after they are off the diet or after six months on a diet. There is no long-term data on the effects of ketosis on kidney function; thus, no complete conclusions can be made. People with preexisting kidney issues are the only ones who get problems from high protein intake. From an unscientific point of view, one would expect increased incidents of this to happen to athletes who consume very high protein diets, but it has not happened. This suggests that high protein intake, under normal conditions, is not harmful to the kidneys. To limit the possibility of kidney stones, it is advised to drink a lot of water to maintain hydration. People who are predisposed to kidney stones should have their kidney function should be monitored to ensure that no complications arise if they decide to follow through with the diet.

Constipation

A common side effect of the diet is reduced bowel movements and constipation. This arises from two different causes: lack of fiber and gastrointestinal absorption of foods. First, the lack of carbs in the diet means that unless supplements are taken, fiber intake is low. Fiber is very important to our systems. High fiber intake can prevent some health conditions, including heart disease and some forms of cancer. Use some type of sugar-free fiber supplement to prevent any health problems and help you maintain regular bowel movements. The diet also reduces the volume of stool due to enhanced absorption and digestion of food; thus, fewer waste products are generated.

Fat regain

Dieting, in general, has very low long term success rates. There are some effects of getting out of a ketogenic diet like the regain of fat lost through calorific restriction alone. This is true for any diet based on calorific restriction. It is expected for weight to be regained after carb reintroduction. For people who use the weighing scale to measure their success, they may completely shun carbs as they think it is the main reason for the weight regain. You should understand that most of the initial weight gain is water and glycogen.

Immune system

There is a large variety in the immunity system response to ketogenic diets on different people. There has been some repost on reduction on some ailments such allergies and increased minor sickness susceptibility.

Optic neuropathy

This is optic nerve dysfunction. It has appeared in a few cases, but it is still existence. It was linked to the people not getting adequate amounts of calcium or vitamin supplements for about a year. All the cases were corrected by supplementation of adequate vitamin B, especially thiamine.

7 tips for success for beginners

Routines are essential on this diet, and it's something that will help you stay healthy. As such, in this phase, we are going to be giving you tips and tricks to make this diet work better for you and help you get an idea of routines that you can put in place for yourself.

Tip number one

DRINK WATER! That is vital for any diet that you're on, and you need it if not on one as well. However, this essential tip is crucial on a keto diet because when you are eating fewer carbs, you are storing less water, meaning that you will get dehydrated very quickly. It would be better if you aimed for more than the daily amount of water; however, think back that drinking too much water can be fatal as your kidneys can only handle so much as once. It has mostly happened to soldiers in the military, it does happen to dieters, so it is something to be aware of.

Tip number two

Do it as a daily routine to try and lower your stress. Stress will not allow you to get into ketosis, which states that keto wants to put you in. The reason for this being that stress increases the hormone known as cortisol in your blood. That is because your body has too much sugar in your blood. If you're dealing with a high level of stress right now, then this diet is not a great idea. Some great ideas for this would be getting into the habit or routine of taking the time to do relaxing activities, such as walking and making sure that sleep well, which leads to another exercise that you need to do.

Tip number three

Staying consistent is another routine that you need to get yourself into. No matter what you are choosing to do, make sure it's something that you can do. Try a routine for a couple of weeks and make serious notes of mental and physical problems that you're going through and any emotional issues that come your way. Make changes as necessary until you find something that works well for you and stick to it. Remember that you need to give yourself time to get used to this and time to get used to changes before giving up.

Tip number four

Be honest with yourself, as well. That is another big tip for this diet. If you're not honest with yourself, this isn't going to work. Another reason you need to be honest with yourself is if something isn't working, you need to understand that and change it. Are you giving yourself enough time to make changes? Are you pushing too hard? If yes, you need to understand what is going on with yourself and how you need to deal with the changes that you're going through. Remember not to get upset or frustrated. This diet takes time, and you need to be a little more patient to make this work effectively.

Tip number five

Getting into the routine of cooking for yourself will also help you so much on this diet. Eating out is fun, but honestly, it can be hard to eat out on this diet. It is practicable to do so with a little bit of special ordering and creativity, but you can avoid all the trouble by only cooking for yourself. It saves time, and it saves a lot of cash.

Get into the habit of cleaning your kitchen. It's tough to stick to a diet if your kitchen is dirty and full of junk food. Clear out the junk and replace all of the wrong food with healthy keto food instead. Remember, with this diet, no soda, pasta, bread, candy, and things. Replacing your food with healthy food and making a routine of cleaning your kitchen and keeping the bad food out will help you be more successful with your diet, which is what you want here.

Tip number six

Another tip is to make sure that you're improving your gut health. That is so important. Your gut is pretty much linked to every other system in your body, so make sure that this something that you want to take seriously.

Tip number seven

The last tip is to mention exercise again. Getting into the exercise routine can boost your ketone levels, and it can help you with your issues on transitioning to keto. Exercises also use different types of energy for your fuel that you need. When your body gets rid of the glycogen storage, it needs other forms of power, and it will turn into that energy that you need. Just remember to avoid exercises that are going to hurt you. Stay in the smaller activities and lower intensity.

Following these tips and getting into these routines will keep you stay on track and make sure that your diet will go as smoothly as possible.

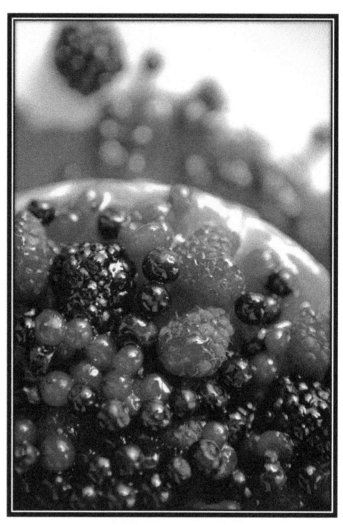

Breakfast

Bacon Cheeseburger Waffles

Preparation Time: 10 Minutes | **Cooking Time:** 20 Minutes | **Servings:** 4

Ingredients

- ❖ Toppings
- ❖ Pepper and Salt to taste
- ❖ 1.5 ounces of cheddar cheese
- ❖ 4 tablespoons of sugar-free barbecue sauce
- ❖ 4 slices of bacon
- ❖ 4 ounces of ground beef, 70% lean meat and 30% fat
- ❖ Waffle dough
- ❖ Pepper and salt to taste
- ❖ 3 tablespoons of parmesan cheese, grated
- ❖ 4 tablespoons of almond flour
- ❖ ¼ teaspoon of onion powder
- ❖ ¼ teaspoon of garlic powder
- ❖ 1 cup (125 g) of cauliflower crumbles
- ❖ 2 large eggs
- ❖ 1.5 ounces of cheddar cheese

Directions

Shred about 3 ounces of cheddar cheese, then add in cauliflower crumbles in a bowl and put in half of the cheddar cheese.

Put into the mixture spices, almond flour, eggs, and parmesan cheese, then mix and put aside for some time.

Thinly slice the bacon and cook in a skillet on medium to high heat.

After the bacon is cooked partially, put in the beef, cook until the mixture is well done.

Then put the excess grease from the bacon mixture into the waffle mixture. Set aside the bacon mix.

Use an immersion blender to blend the waffle mix until it becomes a paste, then add into the waffle iron half of the mix and cook until it becomes crispy.

Repeat for the remaining waffle mixture.

As the waffles cook, add sugar-free barbecue sauce to the ground beef and bacon mixture in the skillet.

Then proceed to assemble waffles by topping them with half of the left cheddar cheese and half the beef mixture. Repeat this for the remaining waffles, broil for around 1-2 minutes until the cheese has melted then serve right away.

Nutrition:

Protein: 18.8grams | Fats: 33.94grams | Calories: 405.25 | Carbohydrates: 4.35grams

Keto Breakfast Cheesecake

Preparation Time: 20 Minutes

Cooking Time: 45 Minutes

Servings: 24 mini cheesecakes

Ingredients

- ❖ Toppings
- ❖ 1/4 cup of mixed berries for each cheesecake, frozen and thawed
- ❖ Filling ingredients
- ❖ 1/2 teaspoon of vanilla extract
- ❖ 1/2 teaspoon of almond extract
- ❖ 3/4 cup of sweetener
- ❖ 6 eggs
- ❖ 8 ounces of cream cheese
- ❖ 16 ounces of cottage cheese
- ❖ Crust ingredients
- ❖ 4 tablespoons of salted butter
- ❖ 2 tablespoons of sweetener
- ❖ 2 cups of almonds, whole

Directions

Preheat oven to around 350 degrees F.

Pulse almonds in a food processor then add in butter and sweetener.

Pulse until all the ingredients mix well and coarse dough forms.

Coat twelve silicone muffin pans using foil or paper liners. Divide the batter evenly between the muffin pans then press into the bottom part until it forms a crust and bakes for about 8 minutes.

In the meantime, mix in a food processor the cream cheese and cottage cheese then pulse until the mixture is smooth. Put in the extracts and sweetener then combine until well mixed.

Add in eggs and pulse again until it becomes smooth; you might need to scrape down the mixture from the sides of the processor. Share equally the batter between the muffin pans, then bake for around 30-40 minutes until the middle is not wobbly when you shake the muffin pan lightly.

Put aside until cooled completely, then put in the refrigerator for about 2 hours and then top with frozen and thawed berries.

Nutrition

Fats: 12g

Calories: 152g

Proteins: 6g

Carbohydrates: 3g

Egg-Crust Pizza

Preparation Time: 5 Minutes

Cooking Time: 15 Minutes

Servings: 1-2

Ingredients

- ❖ ¼ teaspoon of dried oregano to taste
- ❖ ½ teaspoon of spike seasoning to taste
- ❖ 1 ounce of mozzarella, chopped into small cubes
- ❖ 6 – 8 sliced thinly black olives
- ❖ 6 slices of turkey pepperoni, sliced into half
- ❖ 4-5 thinly sliced small grape tomatoes
- ❖ 2 eggs, beaten well
- ❖ 1-2 teaspoons of olive oil

Directions

Preheat the broiler in an oven than in a small bowl, beat well the eggs. Cut the pepperoni and tomatoes in slices then cut the mozzarella cheese into cubes.

Put some olive oil in a skillet over medium heat, then heat the pan for around one minute until it begins to get hot. Add in eggs and season with oregano and spike seasoning, then cook for around 2 minutes until the eggs begin to set at the bottom.

Drizzle half of the mozzarella, olives, pepperoni, and tomatoes on the eggs followed by another layer of the remaining half of the above ingredients. Ensure that there is a lot of cheese on the topmost layers. Cover the skillet using a lid and cook until the cheese begins to melt and the eggs are set, for around 3-4 minutes.

Place the pan under the preheated broiler and cook until the top has browned and the cheese has melted nicely for around 2-3 minutes. Serve immediately.

Nutrition

Calories: 363g

Fats: 24.1g

Carbohydrates: 20.8g

Proteins: 19.25g

Breakfast Roll-Ups

Preparation Time: 5 Minutes

Cooking Time: 15 Minutes

Servings: 5 roll-ups

Ingredients

- ❖ Non-stick cooking spray
- ❖ 5 patties of cooked breakfast sausage
- ❖ 5 slices of cooked bacon
- ❖ 1.5 cups of cheddar cheese, shredded
- ❖ Pepper and salt
- ❖ 10 large eggs

Directions

Preheat a skillet on medium to high heat, then using a whisk, combine two of the eggs in a mixing bowl.

After the pan has become hot, lower the heat to medium-low heat then put in the eggs. If you want to, you can utilize some cooking spray.

Season eggs with some pepper and salt.

Cover the eggs and leave them to cook for a couple of minutes or until the eggs are almost cooked.

Drizzle around 1/3 cup of cheese on top of the eggs, then place a strip of bacon and divide the sausage into two and place on top.

Roll the egg carefully on top of the fillings. The roll-up will almost look like a taquito. If you have a hard time folding over the egg, use a spatula to keep the egg intact until the egg has molded into a roll-up.

Put aside the roll-up then repeat the above steps until you have four more roll-ups; you should have 5 roll-ups in total.

Nutrition:

Calories: 412.2g

Fats: 31.66g

Carbohydrates: 2.26g

Proteins: 28.21g

Basic Opie Rolls

Preparation Time: 20 Minutes

Cooking Time: 35 Minutes

Servings: 12 rolls

Ingredients

- ❖ 1/8 teaspoon of salt
- ❖ 1/8 teaspoon of cream of tartar
- ❖ 3 ounces of cream cheese
- ❖ 3 large eggs

Directions

Preheat the oven to about 300 degrees F, then separate the egg whites from egg yolks and place both eggs in different bowls. Using an electric mixer, beat well the egg whites until the mixture is very bubbly, then add in the cream of tartar and mix again until it forms a stiff peak.

In the bowl with the egg yolks, put in 3 ounces of cubed cheese and salt. Mix well until the mixture has doubled in size and is pale yellow. Put in the egg white mixture into the egg yolk mixture then fold the mixture gently together.

Spray some oil on the cookie sheet coated with some parchment paper, then add dollops of the batter and bake for around 30 minutes.

You will know they are ready when the upper part of the rolls is firm and golden. Leave them to cool for a few minutes on a wire rack. Enjoy with some coffee.

Nutrition:

Calories: 45

Fats: 4g

Carbohydrates: 0g

Proteins: 2g

Almond Coconut Egg Wraps

Preparation time: 5 minutes

Cooking time: 5 minutes

Servings: 4

Ingredients:

- ❖ 5 Organic eggs
- ❖ 1 tbsp Coconut flour
- ❖ 25 tsp Sea salt
- ❖ 2 tbsp almond meal

Directions:

Combine the fixings in a blender and work them until creamy.

Heat a skillet using the med-high temperature setting.

Pour two tablespoons of batter into the skillet and cook -

covered about three minutes. Turn it over to cook for another

3 minutes. Serve the wraps piping hot.

Nutrition:

Carbohydrates: 3 grams

Protein: 8 grams

Fats: 8 grams

Calories: 111

Bacon & Avocado Omelet

Preparation time: 5 minutes

Cooking time: 5 minutes

Servings: 1

Ingredients:

- ❖ 1 slice Crispy bacon
- ❖ 2 Large organic eggs
- ❖ 5 cup freshly grated parmesan cheese
- ❖ 2 tbsp Ghee or coconut oil or butter
- ❖ half of 1 small Avocado

Directions:

Prepare the bacon to your liking and set aside. Combine the eggs, parmesan cheese, and your choice of finely chopped herbs. Warm a skillet and add the butter/ghee to melt using the medium-high heat setting. When the pan is hot, whisk and add the eggs.

Prepare the omelet working it towards the middle of the pan for about 30 seconds. When firm, flip, and cook it for another 30 seconds. Arrange the omelet on a plate and garnish with the crunched bacon bits. Serve with sliced avocado.

Nutrition:

Carbohydrates: 3.3 grams | Protein: 30 grams | Fats: 63 grams | Calories: 719

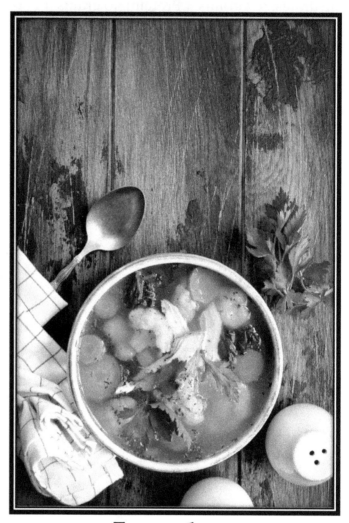

Lunch

Chicken, Bacon and Avocado Cloud Sandwiches

Preparation Time: 10 minutes

Cooking time: 25 minutes

Servings: 6

Ingredients:

- ❖ For cloud bread
- ❖ 3 large eggs
- ❖ 4 oz. cream cheese
- ❖ ½ tablespoon. ground psyllium husk powder
- ❖ ½ teaspoon baking powder
- ❖ A pinch of salt
- ❖ To assemble sandwich
- ❖ 6 slices of bacon, cooked and chopped
- ❖ 6 slices pepper Jack cheese
- ❖ ½ avocado, sliced
- ❖ 1 cup cooked chicken breasts, shredded
- ❖ 3 tablespoons. mayonnaise

Directions:

Preheat your oven to 300 degrees.

Prepare a baking sheet by lining it with parchment paper.

Separate the egg whites and egg yolks, and place into separate bowls.

Whisk the egg whites until very stiff. Set aside.

Combined egg yolks and cream cheese.

Add the psyllium husk powder and baking powder to the egg yolk mixture. Gently fold in.

Add the egg whites into the egg mixture and gently fold in.

Dollop the mixture onto the prepared baking sheet to create 12 cloud bread. Use a spatula to gently spread the circles around to form ½-inch thick pieces.

Bake for 25 minutes or until the tops are golden brown.

Allow the cloud bread to cool completely before serving. It can be refrigerated for up to 3 days or frozen for up to 3 months. If food prepping, place a layer of parchment paper between each bread slice to avoid having them getting stuck together. Simply toast in the oven for 5 minutes when it is time to servings.

To assemble sandwiches, place mayonnaise on one side of one cloud bread. Layer with the remaining sandwich Ingredients: and top with another slice of cloud bread. Servings.

Nutrition:

Calories: 333 kcal

Carbs: 5g

Fat: 26g

Protein: 19.9g

Roasted Lemon Chicken Sandwich

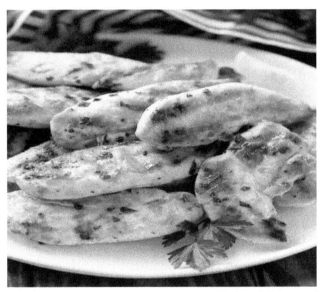

Preparation Time: 15 minutes | **Cooking time:** 1 hour 30 minutes | **Servings:** 12

Ingredients:

- ❖ 1 kg whole chicken
- ❖ 5 tablespoons. butter
- ❖ 1 lemon, cut into wedges
- ❖ 1 tablespoon. garlic powder
- ❖ Salt and pepper to taste
- ❖ 2 tablespoons. mayonnaise
- ❖ Keto-friendly bread

Directions:

Preheat the oven to 350 degrees F.

Grease a deep baking dish with butter.

Ensure that the chicken is patted dry and that the gizzards have been removed.

Combine the butter, garlic powder, salt and pepper.

Rub the entire chicken with it, including in the cavity.

Place the lemon and onion inside the chicken and place the chicken in the prepared baking dish.

Bake for about 1½ hours, depending on the size of the chicken. Baste the chicken often with the drippings. If the drippings begin to dry, add water. The chicken is done when a thermometer insert it into the thickest part of the thigh, reads 165 degrees F or when the clear juices run when the thickest part of the thigh is pierced.

Allow the chicken to cool before slicing.

To assemble the sandwich, shred some of the breast meat and mix with the mayonnaise. Place the mixture between the two bread slices.

To save the chicken, refrigerated for up to 5 days or freeze for up to 1 month.

Nutrition:

Calories: 214 kcal | Carbs: 1.6 g | Fat: 11.8 g | Protein: 24.4 g

Keto-Friendly Skillet Pepperoni Pizza

Preparation Time: 10 minutes

Cooking time: 6 minutes

Servings: 4

Ingredients:

- ❖ For Crust
- ❖ ½ cup almond flour
- ❖ ½ teaspoon baking powder
- ❖ 8 large egg whites, whisked into stiff peaks
- ❖ Salt and pepper to taste
- ❖ Toppings
- ❖ 3 tablespoons. unsweetened tomato sauce
- ❖ ½ cup shredded cheddar cheese
- ❖ ½ cup pepperoni

Directions

Gently incorporate the almond flour into the egg whites.

Ensure that no lumps remain.

Stir in the remaining crust ingredients.

Heat a nonstick skillet over medium heat. Spray with nonstick spray.

Pour the batter into the heated skillet to cover the bottom of the skillet.

Cover the skillet with a lid and cook the pizza crust to cook for about 4 minutes or until bubbles that appear on the top.

Flip the dough and add the toppings, starting with the tomato sauce and ending with the pepperoni

Cook the pizza for 2 more minutes.

Allow the pizza to cool slightly before serving.

It can be stored in the refrigerator for up to 5 days and frozen for up to 1 month.

Nutrition:

Calories: 175 kcal

Carbs: 1.9 g

Fat: 12 g

Protein: 14.3 g

Cheesy Chicken Cauliflower

Preparation Time: 5 minutes | **Cooking time:** 10 minutes | **Servings:** 4

Ingredients:

- ❖ 2 cups cauliflower florets, chopped
- ❖ ½ cup red bell pepper, chopped
- ❖ 1 cup roasted chicken, shredded (Lunch Recipes: Roasted Lemon Chicken Sandwich)
- ❖ ¼ cup shredded cheddar cheese
- ❖ 1 tablespoon. butter
- ❖ 1 tablespoon. sour cream
- ❖ Salt and pepper to taste

Directions:

Stir fry the cauliflower and peppers in the butter over medium heat until the veggies are tender.

Add the chicken and cook until the chicken is warmed through.

Add the remaining **Ingredients:** and stir until the cheese is melted. Serve warm.

Nutrition: Calories: 144 kcal | Carbs: 4 g | Fat: 8.5 g | Protein: 13.2 g

Chicken Soup

Preparation Time: 10 minutes

Cooking time: 25 minutes

Servings: 6

Ingredients:

- ❖ 4 cups roasted chicken, shredded (Lunch Recipes: Roasted Lemon Chicken Sandwich)
- ❖ 2 tablespoons. butter
- ❖ 2 celery stalks, chopped
- ❖ 1 cup mushrooms, sliced
- ❖ 4 cups green cabbage, sliced into strips
- ❖ 2 garlic cloves, minced
- ❖ 6 cups chicken broth
- ❖ 1 carrot, sliced
- ❖ Salt and pepper to taste
- ❖ 1 tablespoon. garlic powder
- ❖ 1 tablespoon. onion powder

Directions:

Sauté the celery, mushrooms and garlic in the butter in a pot over medium heat for 4 minutes.

Add broth, carrots, garlic powder, onion powder, salt, and pepper.

Simmer for 10 minutes or until the vegetables are tender.

Add the chicken and cabbage and simmer for another 10 minutes or until the cabbage is tender.

Servings warm.

It can be refrigerated for up to 3 days or frozen for up to 1 month.

Nutrition:

Calories: 279 kcal

Carbs: 7.5 g

Fat: 12.3 g

Protein: 33.4 g.

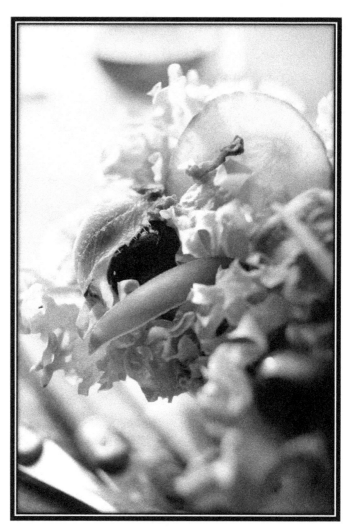

Dinner

Meaty Salad

Preparation Time: 5 minutes

Cooking time: 10

Servings: 2

Ingredients:

- ❖ 3.5 ounces of salami slices
- ❖ 2 cups of spinach
- ❖ A single avocado large and diced
- ❖ 2 tablespoons of olive oil
- ❖ A single teaspoon of balsamic vinegar

Directions:

Toss it all together.

Nutrition:

Calories: 454

Carbs: 10g

Protein: 9g

Fat: 42g

Tomato Salad

Preparation Time: 10 minutes

Cooking time: 5 minutes

Servings: 2

Ingredients:

- ❖ A dozen small spear asparagus
- ❖ 4 raw cherry tomatoes
- ❖ A cup and a half of arugula
- ❖ A single tablespoon of olive oil
- ❖ A tablespoon of whole pieces pine nuts
- ❖ A teaspoon of maple syrup
- ❖ Tablespoon balsamic vinegar
- ❖ 2 tablespoon soft goat cheese

Directions:

Cut the tough ends off asparagus and throw away.

Place the asparagus in a pan of boiling water and cook 3 minutes.

Put in a bowl of ice-cold water right away.

Chill for 60 seconds.

Drain.

Put on a plate.

Slice your tomatoes in half, place on top of the greens.

(arugula and asparagus)

Toss to combine.

Add the nuts to a pan that's dry and on a low heat toast for 2 minutes until it is lightly golden.

Add the syrup and vinegar along with the olive oil to a bowl and whisk, so they combine.

Drizzle the dressing on top and crumble your cheese.

Sprinkle the nuts over the top.

Nutrition:

Calories: 234

Fat: 18g

Protein: 7g

Carbs: 7g

Shrimp with garlic

Preparation Time: 10 min | **Cooking Time:** 25 min |
Servings: 2

Ingredients:

- ❖ 1 lb. shrimp
- ❖ ¼ teaspoon baking soda
- ❖ 2 tablespoons oil
- ❖ 2 teaspoon minced garlic
- ❖ ¼ cup vermouth
- ❖ 2 tablespoons unsalted butter
- ❖ 1 teaspoon parsley

Directions:

In a bowl toss shrimp with baking soda and salt, let it stand for
a couple of minutes

In a skillet heat olive oil and add shrimp

Add garlic, red pepper flakes and cook for 1-2 minutes

Add vermouth and cook for another 4-5 minutes

When ready remove from heat and serve

Nutrition:

Calories: 289 | Total Carbohydrate: 2 g | Cholesterol: 3 mg |
Total Fat: 17 g | Fiber: 2 g | Protein: 7 g | Sodium: 163 mg

Sabich Sandwich

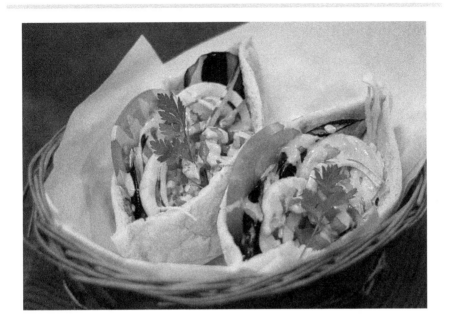

Preparation Time: 5 minutes

Cooking time: 15 minutes

Serving: 2

Ingredients:

- ❖ 2 tomatoes
- ❖ Olive oil
- ❖ ½ lb. eggplant
- ❖ ¼ cucumber
- ❖ 1 tablespoon lemon
- ❖ 1 tablespoon parsley
- ❖ ¼ head cabbage

- ❖ 2 tablespoons wine vinegar
- ❖ 2 pita bread
- ❖ ½ cup hummus
- ❖ ¼ tahini sauce
- ❖ 2 hard-boiled eggs

Directions:

In a skillet fry eggplant slices until tender

In a bowl add tomatoes, cucumber, parsley, lemon juice and season salad

In another bowl toss cabbage with vinegar

In each pita pocket add hummus, eggplant and drizzle tahini sauce

Top with eggs, tahini sauce

Nutrition:

Calories: 289

Total Carbohydrate: 2 g

Cholesterol: 3 mg

Total Fat: 17 g

Fiber: 2 g

Protein: 7 g

Sodium: 163 mg

Salmon with vegetables

Preparation Time: 10 minutes

Cooking time: 15 minutes

Serving: 4

Ingredients:

- ❖ 2 tablespoons olive oil
- ❖ 2 carrots
- ❖ 1 head fennel
- ❖ 2 squash
- ❖ ¼ onion
- ❖ 1-inch ginger
- ❖ 1 cup white wine
- ❖ 2 cups water
- ❖ 2 parsley sprigs
- ❖ 2 tarragon sprigs
- ❖ 6 oz. salmon fillets
- ❖ 1 cup cherry tomatoes
- ❖ 1 scallion

Directions:

In a skillet heat olive oil, add fennel, squash, onion, ginger, carrot and cook until vegetables are soft

Add wine, water, parsley and cook for another 4-5 minutes

Season salmon fillets and place in the pan

Cook for 4-5 minutes per side or until is ready

Transfer salmon to a bowl, spoon tomatoes and scallion around salmon and serve

Nutrition:

Calories: 301

Total Carbohydrate: 2 g

Cholesterol: 13 mg

Total Fat: 17 g

Fiber: 4 g

Protein: 8 g

Sodium: 201 mg

Crispy fish

Preparation Time: 5 minutes |**Cooking time:** 15 minutes | **Serving:** 4

Ingredients:

- ❖ Thick fish fillets
- ❖ ¼ cup all-purpose flour
- ❖ 1 egg
- ❖ 1 cup bread crumbs
- ❖ 2 tablespoons vegetables
- ❖ Lemon wedge

Directions:

In a dish add flour, egg, breadcrumbs in different dishes and set aside

Dip each fish fillet into the flour, egg and then bread crumbs bowl

Place each fish fillet in a heated skillet and cook for 4-5 minutes per side

When ready remove from pan and serve with lemon wedges

Nutrition:

Calories: 189 | Total Carbohydrate: 2 g | Cholesterol: 73 mg | Total Fat: 17 g | Fiber: 0 g | Protein: 7 g | Sodium: 163 mg

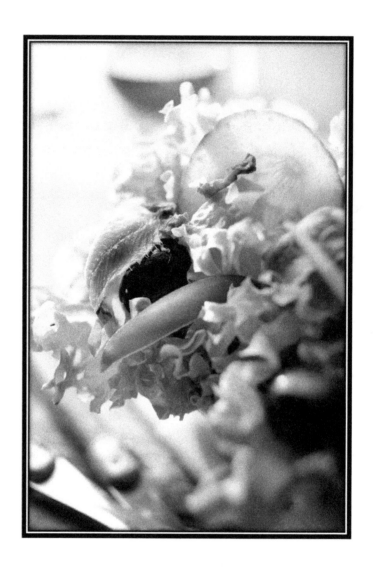

Meat

Beef with Cabbage Noodles

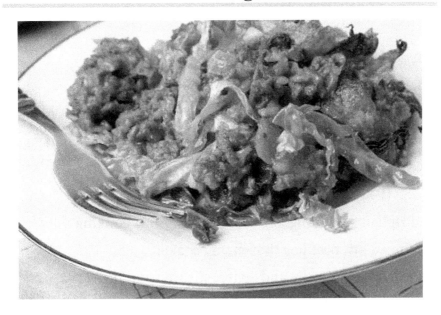

Preparation Time: 5 minutes

Cooking Time: 18 minutes

Servings: 2

Ingredients:

- ❖ 4 oz ground beef
- ❖ 1 cup chopped cabbage
- ❖ 4 oz tomato sauce
- ❖ ½ tsp minced garlic
- ❖ ½ cup of water
- ❖ Seasoning:
- ❖ ½ tbsp coconut oil

- ❖ ½ tsp salt
- ❖ ¼ tsp Italian seasoning
- ❖ 1/8 tsp dried basil

Directions:

Take a skillet pan, place it over medium heat, add oil and when hot, add beef and cook for 5 minutes until nicely browned. Meanwhile, prepare the cabbage and for it slice the cabbage into thin shred.

When the beef has cooked, add garlic, season with salt, basil, and Italian seasoning, stir well and continue cooking for 3 minutes until beef has thoroughly cooked.

Pour in tomato sauce and water, stir well and bring the mixture to boil.

Then reduce heat to medium-low level, add cabbage, stir well until well mixed and simmer for 3 to 5 minutes until cabbage is softened, covering the pan.

Uncover the pan and continue simmering the beef until most of the cooking liquid has evaporated.

Serve.

Nutrition:

188.5 Calories | 12.5 g Fats | 15.5 g Protein | 2.5 g Net Carb | 1 g Fiber

Roast Beef and Mozzarella Plate

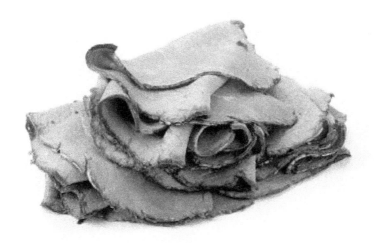

Preparation Time: 5 minutes

Cooking Time: 0 minutes;

Servings: 2

Ingredients:

- ❖ 4 slices of roast beef
- ❖ ½ ounce chopped lettuce
- ❖ 1 avocado, pitted
- ❖ 2 oz mozzarella cheese, cubed
- ❖ ½ cup mayonnaise

- ❖ Seasoning:
- ❖ ¼ tsp salt
- ❖ 1/8 tsp ground black pepper
- ❖ 2 tbsp avocado oil

Directions:

Scoop out flesh from the avocado and divide it evenly between two plates.

Add slices of roast beef, lettuce, and cheese and then sprinkle with salt and black pepper.

Serve with avocado oil and mayonnaise.

Nutrition:

267.7 Calories;

24.5 g Fats;

9.5 g Protein;

1.5 g Net Carb;

2 g Fiber;

Beef and Broccoli

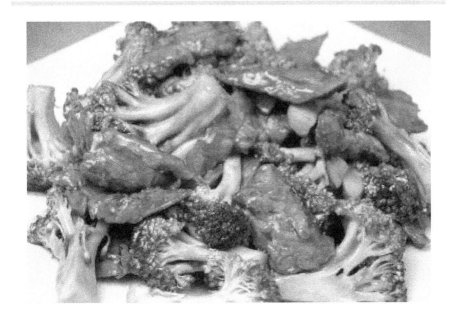

Preparation Time: 5 minutes

Cooking Time: 10 minutes;

Servings: 2

Ingredients:

- ❖ 6 slices of beef roast, cut into strips
- ❖ 1 scallion, chopped
- ❖ 3 oz broccoli florets, chopped
- ❖ 1 tbsp avocado oil
- ❖ 1 tbsp butter, unsalted
- ❖ Seasoning:
- ❖ ¼ tsp salt

- 1/8 tsp ground black pepper
- 1 ½ tbsp soy sauce
- 3 tbsp chicken broth

Directions:

Take a medium skillet pan, place it over medium heat, add oil and when hot, add beef strips and cook for 2 minutes until hot. Transfer beef to a plate, add scallion to the pan, then add butter and cook for 3 minutes until tender.

Add remaining ingredients, stir until mixed, switch heat to the low level and simmer for 3 to 4 minutes until broccoli is tender.

Return beef to the pan, stir until well combined and cook for 1 minute.

Serve.

Nutrition:

245 Calories;

15.7 g Fats;

21.6 g Protein;

1.7 g Net Carb;

1.3 g Fiber;

Garlic Herb Beef Roast

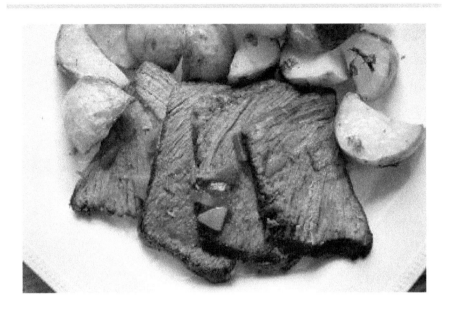

Preparation Time: 5 minutes

Cooking Time: 10 minutes;

Servings: 2

Ingredients:

- ❖ 6 slices of beef roast
- ❖ ½ tsp garlic powder
- ❖ 1/3 tsp dried thyme
- ❖ ¼ tsp dried rosemary
- ❖ 2 tbsp butter, unsalted
- ❖ Seasoning:
- ❖ 1/3 tsp salt

❖ 1/4 tsp ground black pepper

Directions:

Prepare the spice mix and for this, take a small bowl, place garlic powder, thyme, rosemary, salt, and black pepper and then stir until mixed.

Sprinkle spice mix on the beef roast.

Take a medium skillet pan, place it over medium heat, add butter and when it melts, add beef roast and then cook for 5 to 8 minutes until golden brown and cooked.

Serve.

Nutrition:

140 Calories;

12.7 g Fats;

5.5 g Protein;

0.1 g Net Carb;

0.2 g Fiber;

Sprouts Stir-fry with Kale, Broccoli, and Beef

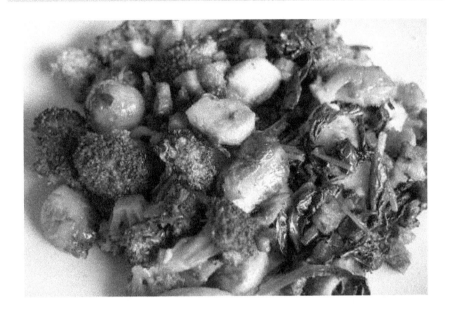

Preparation Time: 5 minutes

Cooking Time: 8 minutes;

Servings: 2

Ingredients:

- ❖ 3 slices of beef roast, chopped
- ❖ 2 oz Brussels sprouts, halved
- ❖ 4 oz broccoli florets
- ❖ 3 oz kale
- ❖ 1 ½ tbsp butter, unsalted
- ❖ 1/8 tsp red pepper flakes
- ❖ Seasoning:

- ❖ ¼ tsp garlic powder
- ❖ ¼ tsp salt
- ❖ 1/8 tsp ground black pepper

Directions:

Take a medium skillet pan, place it over medium heat, add ¾ tbsp butter and when it melts, add broccoli florets and sprouts, sprinkle with garlic powder, and cook for 2 minutes.

Season vegetables with salt and red pepper flakes, add chopped beef, stir until mixed and continue cooking for 3 minutes until browned on one side.

Then add kale along with remaining butter, flip the vegetables and cook for 2 minutes until kale leaves wilts.

Serve.

Nutrition:

125 Calories;

9.4 g Fats;

4.8 g Protein;

1.7 g Net Carb;

2.6 g Fiber;

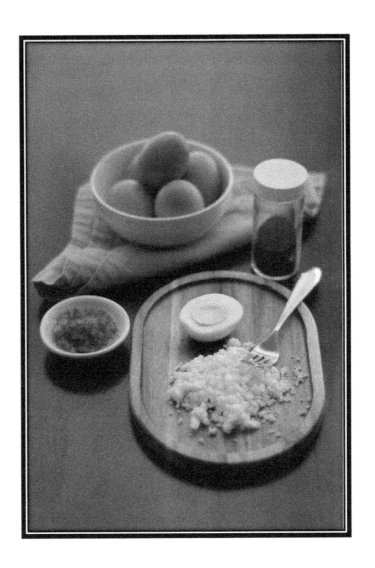

Poultry

Egg Butter

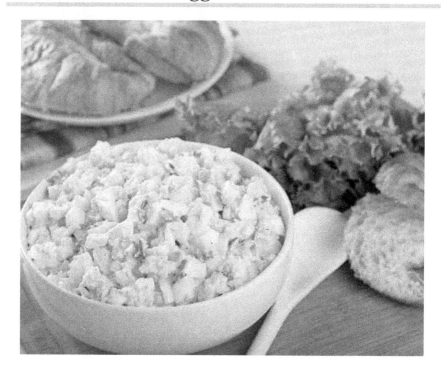

Preparation Time: 5 minutes;

Cooking Time: 0 minutes;

Servings: 2

Ingredients:

- ❖ 2 large eggs, hard-boiled
- ❖ 3-ounce unsalted butter
- ❖ ½ tsp dried oregano
- ❖ ½ tsp dried basil
- ❖ 2 leaves of iceberg lettuce

- ❖ Seasoning:
- ❖ ½ tsp of sea salt
- ❖ ¼ tsp ground black pepper

Directions:

Peel the eggs, then chop them finely and place in a medium bowl.

Add remaining Ingredients: and stir well.

Serve egg butter wrapped in a lettuce leaf.

Nutrition:

159 Calories;

Fats; 3 g

Protein; 0.2 g

Net Carb; 0 g

Omelet

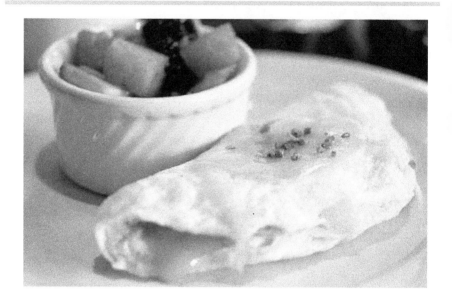

Preparation Time: 5 minutes

Cooking Time: 10 minutes;

Servings: 2

Ingredients:

- ❖ 2 eggs
- ❖ 2 tbsp shredded parmesan cheese, divided
- ❖ 1 tbsp unsalted butter
- ❖ 2 slices of turkey bacon, diced
- ❖ Seasoning:
- ❖ ¼ tsp salt
- ❖ 1/8 tsp ground black pepper

Directions:

Crack eggs in a bowl, add salt and black pepper, whisk well until fluffy and then whisk in 1 tbsp cheese until combined. Take a medium skillet pan, add bacon slices on it, cook for 3 minutes until sauté, then pour in the egg mixture and cook for 4 minutes or until the omelet is almost firm.

Lower heat to medium-low level, sprinkle remaining cheese on top of the omelet, then fold the omelet and cook for 1 minute. Slide the omelet to a plate, cut it in half, and serve immediately.

Nutrition:

114.5 Calories;

9.3 g Fats;

4 g Protein;

1 g Net Carb;

0.2 g Fiber;

Classic Deviled Eggs

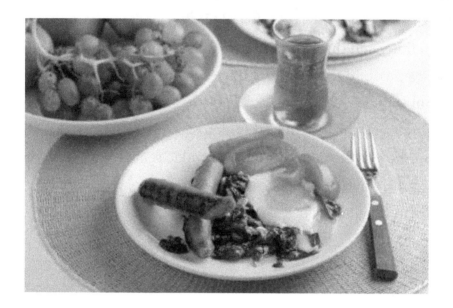

Preparation Time: 5 minutes

Cooking Time: 0 minutes;

Servings: 2

Ingredients:

- ❖ 2 eggs, boiled
- ❖ 1 1/3 tbsp mayonnaise
- ❖ 1/3 tsp mustard paste
- ❖ ¼ tsp apple cider vinegar
- ❖ 1/8 tsp paprika
- ❖ Seasoning:
- ❖ 1/8 tsp salt

❖ 1/8 tsp ground black pepper

Directions:

Peel the boiled eggs, then slice in half lengthwise and transfer egg yolks to a medium bowl by using a spoon.

Mash the egg yolk, add remaining ingredients except for paprika and stir until well combined.

Pipe the egg yolk mixture into egg whites, then sprinkle with paprika and serve.

Nutrition: 145 Calories;

12.8 g Fats;

6.9 g Protein;

0.7 g Net Carb;

0.1 g Fiber;

Green Buttered Eggs

Preparation Time: 5 minutes

Cooking Time: 5 minutes;

Servings: 2

Ingredients:

- ❖ ¼ cup cilantro leaves, chopped
- ❖ 1/2 tsp minced garlic
- ❖ ¼ cup parsley, chopped
- ❖ 1 tsp thyme leaves
- ❖ 2 eggs
- ❖ Seasoning:
- ❖ ¼ tsp salt
- ❖ ¼ tsp cayenne pepper
- ❖ 1 tbsp butter, unsalted
- ❖ 1/2 tbsp avocado oil

Directions:

Take a medium skillet pan, place it over low heat, add oil and butter, and when the butter melts, add garlic and cook for 1 minute until fragrant.

Add thyme, cook for 30 seconds until it begins to brown, then add cilantro and parsley, switch heat to medium level and then cook for 2 minutes until crisp.

Cracks eggs on top of herbs, cover with a lid, then switch heat to the low level and cook for 2 to 3 minutes until yolks are set and cooked to the desired level.

Serve.

Nutrition:

165 Calories;

14.4 g Fats;

7.3 g Protein;

0.9 g Net Carb;

0.4 g Fiber;

Egg Salad

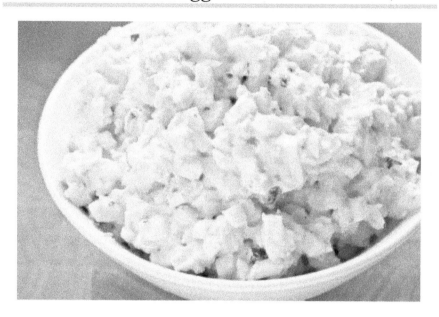

Preparation Time: 5 minutes

Cooking Time: 0 minutes

Servings: 2

Ingredients:

- ❖ 2 tbsp mayonnaise
- ❖ 1 tsp lemon juice
- ❖ 2 large eggs, hard-boiled
- ❖ 2 slices of bacon, cooked, crumbled
- ❖ Seasoning:
- ❖ 1/8 tsp cracked black pepper
- ❖ ¼ tsp salt

Directions:

Peel the eggs, then dice them and place them in a bowl.

Add remaining ingredients except for bacon and stir until well mixed.

Top with bacon and serve.

Nutrition:

240.3 Calories;

10g Fats;

10.8 g Protein;

0 g Net Carb;

0 g Fiber;

Pesto Scramble

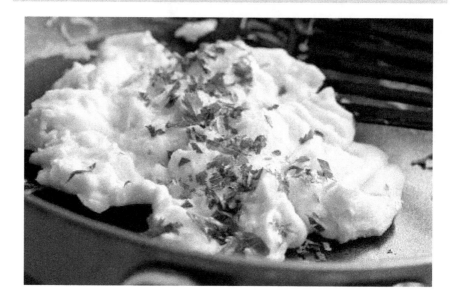

Preparation Time: 5 minutes

Cooking Time: 5 minutes

Servings: 2

Ingredients:

- ❖ 2 eggs
- ❖ 2 tbsp grated cheddar cheese
- ❖ 1 tbsp unsalted butter
- ❖ 1 tbsp basil pesto
- ❖ Seasoning:
- ❖ 1/8 tsp salt
- ❖ 1/8 tsp ground black pepper

Directions:

Crack eggs in a bowl, add cheese, black pepper, salt, and pesto and whisk until combined.

Take a skillet pan, place it over medium heat, add butter and when it melts, pour in the egg mixture, and cook for 3 to 5 minutes until eggs have scrambled to the desired level.

Serve.

Nutrition:

159.5 Calories;

14.5 g Fats;

7 g Protein;

0.4 g Net Carb;

0.1 g Fiber;

Fried Eggs

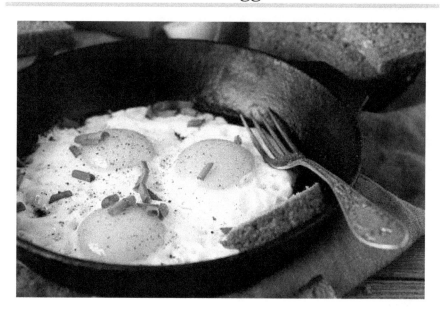

Preparation Time: 5 minutes

Cooking Time: 8 minutes

Servings: 2

Ingredients:

- ❖ 2 eggs
- ❖ 2 tbsp unsalted butter
- ❖ Seasoning:
- ❖ ¼ tsp salt
- ❖ 1/8 tsp ground black pepper

Directions:

Take a skillet pan, place it over medium heat, add butter and when it has melted, crack eggs in the pan.

Cook eggs for 3 to 5 minutes until fried to the desired level, then transfer the eggs to serving plates and sprinkle with salt and black pepper.

Serve.

Nutrition:

179 Calories;

16.5 g Fats;

7.6 g Protein;

0 g Net Carb;

0 g Fiber;

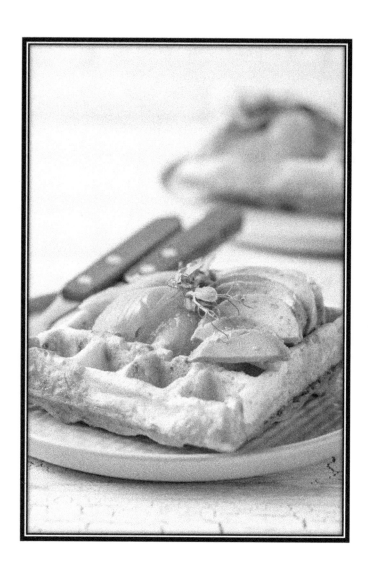

Snacks

Fluffy Bites

Preparation Time: 20 minutes | **Cooking Time:** 60 minutes | **Servings:** 12

Ingredients:

- ❖ 2 Teaspoons Cinnamon
- ❖ 2/3 Cup Sour Cream
- ❖ 2 Cups Heavy Cream
- ❖ 1 Teaspoon Scraped Vanilla Bean
- ❖ ¼ Teaspoon Cardamom
- ❖ 4 Egg Yolks
- ❖ Stevia to Taste

Directions:

Start by whisking your egg yolks until creamy and smooth.

Get out a double boiler, and add your eggs with the rest of your ingredients. Mix well.

Remove from heat, allowing it to cool until it reaches room temperature.

Refrigerate for an hour before whisking well.

Pour into molds, and freeze for at least an hour before serving.

Nutrition:

Calories: 363 | Protein: 2 | Fat: 40 | Carbohydrates: 1

Coconut Fudge

Preparation Time: 20 minutes | **Cooking Time:** 60 minutes |**Servings:** 12

Ingredients:

- ❖ 2 Cups Coconut Oil
- ❖ ½ Cup Dark Cocoa Powder
- ❖ ½ Cup Coconut Cream
- ❖ ¼ Cup Almonds, Chopped
- ❖ ¼ Cup Coconut, Shredded
- ❖ 1 Teaspoon Almond Extract
- ❖ Pinch of Salt
- ❖ Stevia to Taste

Directions:

Pour your coconut oil and coconut cream in a bowl, whisking with an electric beater until smooth. Once the mixture becomes smooth and glossy, do not continue.

Begin to add in your cocoa powder while mixing slowly, making sure that there aren't any lumps.

Add in the rest of your ingredients, and mix well.

Line a bread pan with parchment paper, and freeze until it sets. Slice into squares before serving.

Nutrition:

Calories: 172 | Fat: 20 | Carbohydrates: 3

Nutmeg Nougat

Preparation Time: 30 minutes

Cooking Time: 60 minutes

Servings: 12

Ingredients:

- ❖ 1 Cup Heavy Cream
- ❖ 1 Cup Cashew Butter
- ❖ 1 Cup Coconut, Shredded
- ❖ ½ Teaspoon Nutmeg
- ❖ 1 Teaspoon Vanilla Extract, Pure
- ❖ Stevia to Taste

Directions:

Melt your cashew butter using a double boiler, and then stir in your vanilla extract, dairy cream, nutmeg and stevia. Make sure it's mixed well.

Remove from heat, allowing it to cool down before refrigerating it for a half-hour.

Shape into balls, and coat with shredded coconut. Chill for at least two hours before serving.

Nutrition:

Calories: 341 | Fat: 34 |Carbohydrates: 5

Sweet Almond Bites

Preparation Time: 30 minutes

Cooking Time: 90 minutes

Servings: 12

Ingredients:

- ❖ 18 Ounces Butter, Grass-Fed
- ❖ 2 Ounces Heavy Cream
- ❖ ½ Cup Stevia
- ❖ 2/3 Cup Cocoa Powder
- ❖ 1 Teaspoon Vanilla Extract, Pure
- ❖ 4 Tablespoons Almond Butter

Directions:

Use a double boiler to melt your butter before adding in all of your remaining ingredients.

Place the mixture into molds, freezing for two hours before serving.

Nutrition:

Calories: 350

Protein: 2

Fat: 38

Strawberry Cheesecake Minis

Preparation Time: 30 minutes

Cooking Time: 120 minutes

Servings: 12

Ingredients:

- ❖ 1 Cup Coconut Oil
- ❖ 1 Cup Coconut Butter
- ❖ ½ Cup Strawberries, Sliced
- ❖ ½ Teaspoon Lime Juice
- ❖ 2 Tablespoons Cream Cheese, Full Fat
- ❖ Stevia to Taste

Directions:

Blend your strawberries together.

Soften your cream cheese, and then add in your coconut butter.

Combine all ingredients together, and then pour your mixture into silicone molds.

Freeze for at least two hours before serving.

Nutrition:

Calories: 372 | Protein: 1 | Fat: 41 | Carbohydrates: 2

Cocoa Brownies

Preparation Time: 10 minutes | **Cooking Time:** 30 minutes | **Servings:** 12

Ingredients:

- ❖ 1 Egg
- ❖ 2 Tablespoons Butter, Grass Fed
- ❖ 2 Teaspoons Vanilla Extract, Pure
- ❖ ¼ Teaspoon Baking Powder
- ❖ ¼ Cup Cocoa Powder
- ❖ 1/3 Cup Heavy Cream
- ❖ ¾ Cup Almond Butter
- ❖ Pinch Sea Salt

Directions:

Break your egg into a bowl, whisking until smooth.

Add in all of your wet ingredients, mixing well.

Mix all dry ingredients into a bowl.

Sift your dry ingredients into your wet ingredients, mixing to form a batter.

Get out a baking pan, greasing it before pouring in your mixture.

Heat your oven to 350 and bake for twenty-five minutes.

Allow it to cool before slicing and serve room temperature or warm.

Nutrition:

Calories: 184 | Protein: 1 | Fat: 20 | Carbohydrates: 1

Chocolate Orange Bites

Preparation Time: 20 minutes

Cooking Time: 120 minutes

Servings: 6

Ingredients:

- ❖ 10 Ounces Coconut Oil
- ❖ 4 Tablespoons Cocoa Powder
- ❖ ¼ Teaspoon Blood Orange Extract
- ❖ Stevia to Taste

Directions:

Melt half of your coconut oil using a double boiler, and then add in your stevia and orange extract.

Get out candy molds, pouring the mixture into it. Fill each mold halfway, and then place in the fridge until they set.

Melt the other half of your coconut oil, stirring in your cocoa powder and stevia, making sure that the mixture is smooth with no lumps.

Pour into your molds, filling them up all the way, and then allow it to set in the fridge before serving.

Nutrition:

Calories: *188* | Protein: *1* | Fat: 21 | Carbohydrates: 5

Caramel Cones

Preparation Time: 25 minutes

Cooking Time: 120 minutes

Servings: 6

Ingredients:

- ❖ 2 Tablespoons Heavy Whipping Cream
- ❖ 2 Tablespoons Sour Cream
- ❖ 1 Tablespoon Caramel Sugar
- ❖ 1 Teaspoon Sea Salt, Fine
- ❖ 1/3 Cup Butter, Grass-Fed
- ❖ 1/3 Cup Coconut Oil
- ❖ Stevia to Taste

Directions:

Soften your coconut oil and butter, mixing together.

Mix all ingredients together to form a batter, and then place them in molds.

Top with a little salt, and keep refrigerated until serving.

Nutrition:

Calories: *100*

Fat: 12 Grams

Carbohydrates: 1

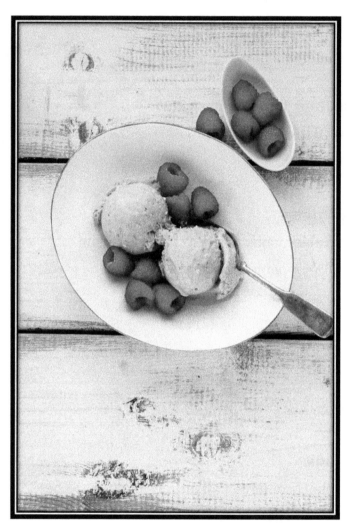

Dessert

Keto and dairy-free vanilla custard

Preparation Time: 11 minutes

Cooking time: 5 minutes

Servings: 4

Ingredients:

- ❖ 6 egg yolks
- ❖ ½ cup unsweetened almond milk
- ❖ 1 tsp vanilla extract
- ❖ ¼ cup melted coconut oil

Directions:

Mix egg yolks, almond milk, vanilla in a metal bowl.

Gradually stir in the melted coconut oil.

Boil water in a saucepan, place the mixing bowl over the saucepan.

Whisk the mixture constantly and vigorously until thickened for about 5 minutes.

. Remover from the saucepan, serve hot or chill in the fridge.

Nutrition:

215.38 Calories | 21g Fats | 1g Carbohydrates | 4g Protein

Keto Triple Chocolate Mug Cake

Preparation Time: 3 minutes | **Cooking time:** 1 minute | **Servings:** 3

Ingredients:

- 1 1/2 tbsp coconut flour
- 1/2 tsp baking powder
- 2 tbsp cacao powder
- 2 tbsp powdered sweetener
- 1 egg medium
- 5 tbsp double/heavy cream
- 2 tbsp sugar-free chocolate chips
- 1/4 tsp vanilla extract optional

Directions:

Mix all dry fixing- coconut flour, baking powder, cacao powder, and a bowl.

Whisk together the egg, cream, and vanilla extract, pour the mixture in the dry ingredients.

Add the chocolate chips in the mixture and let the batter rest for a minute.

Grease the ramekins with the melted butter, pour the batter in the ramekins.

Place in the microwave and microwave for 1 ½ minute until cooked through.

Nutrition:

Calories: 250 | Carbohydrates: 9.7g | Protein: 6g | Fat: 22g

Keto Cheesecake Stuffed Brownies

Preparation Time: 11 minutes

Cooking time: 30 minutes

Servings: 16

Ingredients:

- ❖ For the Filling
- ❖ 8 oz (225g) cream cheese
- ❖ 1/4 cup sweetener
- ❖ 1 large egg
- ❖ For the Brownie
- ❖ 3 oz (85g) low carb milk chocolate
- ❖ 5 tbsp butter
- ❖ 3 large eggs
- ❖ 1/2 cup sweetener
- ❖ 1/4 cup cocoa powder
- ❖ 1/2 cup almond flour

Directions:

Heat-up oven to 350 °F, line a brownie pan with parchment.

In a mixing bowl, whisk together cream cheese, egg, and sweetener until smooth, set aside.

Place chocolate and butter in a microwave-safe bowl and microwave at 30 seconds interval.

Whisk frequently until smooth, allow to cool for a few minutes. Whisk together the remaining eggs and sweetener until fluffy. Mix in the almond flour plus cocoa powder until soft peaks form.

Mix in the chocolate and butter mixture and beat with a hand mixer for a few seconds.

Fill the prepared pan with ¾ of the batter, then top with the cream cheese and the brownie batter. Bake the cheesecake brownie until mostly set for about 25-30 minutes.

The jiggling parts of the cake will firm when you remove it from the oven.

Nutrition:

143.94 Calories

13.48g Fat

1.9g Carbohydrates

3.87g Protein

Keto Raspberry Ice Cream

Preparation Time: 45 minutes

Cooking time: 0 minutes

Servings: 8

Ingredients:

2 cups heavy whipping cream

1 cup raspberries

1/2 cup powdered erythritol

1 pasteurized egg yolk

Directions:

Process all the ice cream ingredients in a food processor.

Add blended mixture into the ice cream maker.

Turn on the ice cream machine and churn according to the manufacturer's directions.

Nutrition:

120 Calories

23g Fats

4g Carbohydrates

0g Protein

Chocolate Macadamia Nut Fat Bombs

Preparation Time: 11 minutes

Cooking time: 30 minutes

Servings: 4

Ingredients:

- 1⅓ oz (38g) sugar-free dark chocolate
- 1 tbsp coconut oil
- coarse salt or sea salt
- 1½ oz (42g) raw macadamia nuts halves

Directions:

Put three macadamia nut halves in each of 8 wells of the mini muffin pan.

Microwave the chocolate chips for about a few seconds.

Whisk until smooth, add coconut oil and salt, mix until well combined.

Fill the mini muffin pan with the chocolate mixture to cover the nuts completely.

Refrigerate the muffin pan until chilled and firm for about 30 minutes.

Nutrition:

153 Calories | 1 Fat | 2g Carbohydrates | 4g Protein

Keto Peanut Butter Chocolate Bars

Preparation Time: 11 minutes | **Cooking time:** 10 minutes | **Servings:** 8

Ingredients:

- For the Bars
- 3/4 cup (84 g) Superfine Almond Flour
- 2 oz (56.7 g) Butter
- 1/4 cup (45.5 g) Swerve, Icing sugar style
- 1/2 cup Peanut Butter
- 1 tsp Vanilla extract
- For the Topping
- 1/2 cup (90 g) Sugar-Free Chocolate Chips

Directions:

Combine all the ingredients for the bars and spread into a small 6-inch pan.

Microwave the chocolate in the microwave oven for 30 seconds and whisk until smooth.

Pour the melted chocolate in over the bars ingredients.

Refrigerate for at least an hour or two until the bars firmed.

Keep in an airtight container.

Nutrition:

246 Calories | 23g Fats | 7g Carbohydrates | 7g Protein

Salted Toffee Nut Cups

Preparation Time: 11 minutes | **Cooking time:** 10 minutes | **Servings:** 5

Ingredients:

- 5 oz (141g) low-carb milk chocolate
- 3 tbsp + 2 tbsp sweetener
- 3 tbsp cold butter
- ½ oz (14g) raw walnuts, chopped
- Sea salt to taste

Directions:

Microwave the chocolate in 45 seconds intervals and continue whisk until chocolate melted.

Line the cupcake pan with 5 paper liners and add chocolate to the bottom of the cupcake.

Spread the chocolate to coat the bottom of the cupcake evenly, freeze to harden.

In a heat-proof bowl, heat the cold butter and sweetener on power 8 for three minutes.

Stir the butter every 20 seconds to prevent the burning.

Mix in the 2 tbsp of sweetener and whisk to thicken. Fold in the walnuts.

Fill the chocolate cups with the toffee mixture quickly.

Top the cupcakes with the remaining chocolate and refrigerate to firm for 20-30 minutes.

Remove from the cups and sprinkle with sea salt!

Nutrition:

194 Calories

18 g Fat

2 g Carbohydrates

2.5 g Protein

Conclusion

The ketogenic diet is one that has many important aspects and information that you need to know as someone who wants to try this diet. It is important to remember the warning that we have given you at the beginning of the book that this is not a diet that is safe and that doctors recommend you don't try it, or if you are going to attempt it remember that you shouldn't do so for longer than six months and even then never without the constant supervision of a doctor or at the very least a doctor knowing that you're doing this and you following their guidelines and words exactly so that they can make sure that you are safe.

The ketogenic diet is a diet that believes that by minimizing your carbs, you will, while maximizing the good fat in your system and making sure that you're getting the protein you need, that you will be happier and healthier. In this book, we give you the information to know what this diet is all about, as well as describing the different types and areas that this diet will offer. Most people assume that there is only one way to do this, and while there is one thing that the additional options share, there are actually four different options you can choose from. Each one has it's unique benefits, and you should know about each type to learn what would be best for your body, which is why we have described them in the book for you to have the best information possible when you begin this diet for yourself.

Another big thing about this diet is that many people don't understand the importance of exercise with this diet. The best way to become healthier is to do three things for yourself. Get the right amount of sleep, eat healthily, and make sure that you get the proper amount of exercise as well for your body to work at an optimum level. As such, we explain the exercises that are the best to go with your diet to make sure that you are getting the most out of it.

For women who are on the go and have a busy lifestyle, we have provided recipes for a thirty-day meal plan so that you can make food quickly and have a great meal for your lifestyle. They also have enough servings for you to have leftovers so that you don't have to worry about preparing in the morning. Instead, you can simply pack it up and take it with you wherever you go. This works out so much easier for so many people because they don't have to cook in the morning, and it saves a busy person a lot of time.

We also provide helpful ideas on how you can use these recipes for meals to make sure that you see how the numbers will affect you and make an impact on your day. A great example that we have explained is if you have a big breakfast that is full of the protein you need, for example, thirty grams, you've got to take note of this and be aware because if you eat too much for your dinner or another meal, you will throw your numbers out of where they are supposed to be. For those that have more time on their hands, we offer a thirty-day meal plan for you as well with all-new recipes to enjoy and tips and tricks for making them work for you in the best way.

With all of this information at your fingertips, you will be able to enjoy this diet and use it to your advantage. Another benefit that we offer? We explain routines that you can do for yourself to make this diet last longer for you and to benefit your body better as a result. Routines are very important and can be a big help to your body but also your spirit and your mind. This will help you utilize the diet better, and you will be able to improve with it as well as have it become easier for you to handle.

As many people are using this diet to their benefit, knowing your food is one of the biggest parts of this, and it becomes easier once you begin to use this in your daily life. One of the best things you can do is pay attention to the food that your eating and how it affects your body and mind. You will notice that this diet has the ability to make you sick, which isn't a good thing, and it's one of the things the doctors warn against. For this reason, it's very important to pay attention to what your eating and how your feeling at the same time. Another warning that we have said you need to pay attention to is that you will need to make sure that your ketogenic 'flu' isn't the result of something more serious. As people are being told that this is normal, this book has brought you the knowledge you need to be able to tell you why it's not.

This book has given you all the information you need to do this diet properly and to do it well. It's important to understand what you're getting into when you go into this diet, and this book will give you valuable information that you can use to your benefit and so you can avoid the problems that can come with this diet. You want to stay healthy and make sure that your body is able to do what it needs to. As with anything, we have put a strong emphasis on the fact that if anything feels wrong or unnatural, you will need to see a doctor to make sure that you are safe and that your body can handle this diet. Use the knowledge in this book to have amazing recipes and learn directions for amazing meals for yourself.

CPSIA information can be obtained
at www.ICGtesting.com
Printed in the USA
BVHW041010150321
602551BV00006B/384